Also by Dr. Stenbeck

Available from the usual on-line source

Books
Healing Yourself -- The Holistic Approach
  [An introduction to Holistic Self-healing.]

Heal Yourself Right Now!
  *[The Seven Priority Organ Levels for
  effective Nutritional/Holistic Treatment of
  all organs.]*

The 22 Unique Body Types
  (for Health and Weight Loss)

Q & A to Identify Your Body Type (Booklet)
  [Individual Type booklets are also available]

Booklets
(Step-by-step instructions on healing yourself)

  #1 Start Healing with Positive Thinking
  #2 Mastering Positive Feelings for Health!
  #3 Spiritual Balance and Your Healing

Q & A
to Identify your Body Type

for Health and Weight Loss

Know the mineral and nutritional healing needs for your individuality, your health challenges, stress management, success spheres, personality strengths and weaknesses, and more...

For Kaye,
there at the beginning with Doc Severn,
and for Liberty,
continuing the holistic healing journey…

Disclaimer

The information in this booklet is for educational purposes only and is not a substitute for medication, diets, or other medical care. The diets do not treat diseases or medical conditions, and are an adjunct to your orthodox health care.

The author and publisher accept no responsibility for any misuse of the information within. If you have any physical problem, food allergy, emotional disorder, or disease, common sense dictates that you consult with a physician before changing your diet, taking nutritional supplements, or following the advice given here.

———

About the Author

Educated in New Zealand and in the U.S.A., Dr. Stenbeck attained B.Sc. (NZ), M.S., and D.C. degrees. His holistic healing methods have been profiled in magazines (Esquire, McLean's, Playgirl, the Atlanta Constitution), and on TV in the USA and in Canada. He was the main contributor to the Warner Book, _The Eye/Body Connection_ by Jessica Maxwell that focused on the holistic healing relationships between the iris structure and organ genetics.

In the 1970-80's he was elected Fellow, Royal Society of Health, London; Fellow, American Association of Chemists; Member, American Association of Clinical Chemists; and Affiliate, Royal Society of Medicine, London. He studied naturopathy and Body Types with Dr. Bernard Jensen and Dr. Clifford Severn, and has practiced in medical partnerships where patients received the joint benefits of medical and holistic healing.

He is a member of Self-Realization Fellowship. To receive advice on any health issue from a holistic viewpoint, or to receive help with your body type, see his web site: *DrStenbeck.net*

———

Contents

1. *Identify your Probable Type Class*

Identify your Type Class:
Thin, Muscle, or Fat   *1*

2. *The 6 Thin Types*   *13*
(Identify Your Brief Type Description)

Atrophic, Exesthesic, Marasmic,
Neurogenic, Pathoferic, Sillevitic

3. *The 9 Muscle Types*   *27*
(Identify Your Brief Type Description)

Calciferic, Carbogenic, Desmogenic,
Eldic, Medeic, Myogenic, Nervimotive,
Nitropheric, Pallinomic

Succinct Quote on Human Types

From Victor Rocine, who first described discrete body types around 1900.

"A type is an order of people that differentiates and distinguishes itself by a general and similar form, brain-formation, chemistry, structure, build, immunity, tendencies, predisposition, resemblance, skin-pigment, and type characteristics based on observation and analogy.

"Or, in other words, people of a given type are similar physically and like-minded as if they were brothers and sisters—that is what type means.

"Everything in nature is made according to plan. Man only discovers that plan and gives it a name. The zoologist has not made the animals—he has only described the plan adopted by the wonderful Creator, and named the classes, sub-classes, etc.

"How important type research will be to humanity, time alone will make known."

———

Brief Extract from "The 22 Unique Body Types"

Introduction

Type comes from 'typus' meaning an image or impression, the study of types being called typology.

▶ *Rocine: "A combination of mental and structural features is consistently found in people of the same type."*

Rocine wrote that all types are a mixture of positive and negative qualities. He based his work on the biochemical individuality of our *mineral* absorption and utilization. Of course, all minerals are absorbed, but he postulated that different types of people *selectively* absorb certain minerals, to a greater or lesser extent, requiring specific mineral foods for their enhanced health and healing. This is the basis of his types.

▶ *The type information cannot predict what or who you will become, or how successful or not, but your type is capable of bringing a creative excellence to whatever you do in life. If your type has negative qualities that you disagree with, remember that they are only tendencies and may or may not manifest in you.*

This book enlarges on Rocine's premise (early 1900's), along with my fifty years of observations and experience with this subject, and integrated with the later research of Herbert Sheldon, M.D., Ph.D., at Harvard University (1930's) who utilized these terms:

Ectomorph (Thin Types)
Mesomorph (Muscle Types)
Endomorph (Fat Types).

Comparing your shared physical (and sometimes psychological) descriptions with the Celebrity Lists further assists the identification of your type. It is not that you will look exactly like, or be a twin to, any particular celebrity. Look closely at a celebrity's features: face, profile, height, weight, head, etc. If you know something about their talents, beliefs, success and failure spheres, health and weight challenges, attitudes and behaviors, etc., then you get clues as to what your type may be.

———

Understanding Types and Sub-Types

Each of us has a clearly discernible dominant type. Visualize the celebrity examples from movies, politics, sports, the arts and public life, and try to identify with their physical features. Look for similar features, remembering that you will not recognize all attributes in yourself. You are not looking for your twin!

The sub-type issue is the main reason people of the same major type can look so different. Remember that a type description does not characterize you exactly, but depicts your individual variant of a type.

———

Minerals

Minerals are essential life nutrients that accelerate enzyme and chemical reactions and provide a basis for your body typing. Although found in all tissues, different minerals tend to be concentrated in certain organs, their presence or absence contributing to the healing of such tissues; e.g., zinc accelerates prostate healing; calcium and manganese promote bone, joint and connective tissue healing.

Specific foods nurture each type, some people needing meats for their health others needing a vegetarian diet. A high potassium diet nurtures one person, while another needs high sulfur, calcium, zinc, or another mineral.

Mineral Digestion and Absorption

Compared to vitamins, minerals are *difficult* to digest, absorb, and utilize. In people with strong digestive systems, this aspect may not be important. The following factors should be in place for optimal mineral metabolism:

1. Stomach Hydrochloric Acid Production
2. Parathyroid Hormone Balance
3. Organ Toxic Metal and Chemical Removal

Total Body Healing

Note that from a holistic healing perspective, in addition to minerals and type information, the following healing factors are necessary:

> *Nutrient Balance*
> *Mental Balance*
> *Emotional Balance*
> *Spiritual Balance*
> *Detoxifying Integrity*

The above factors are all important to your total healing especially if you are interested in self-healing (see my earlier book, <u>Healing Yourself</u>).

———

―――――

This Booklet is for those people desiring to first identify their body type, before obtaining The 22 Unique Body Types, or the appropriate type booklet. The Questionnaires are not foolproof and you may need to read all the type descriptions in detail, to determine your type.

―――――

1

Identify Your Probable Type Class

(Thin, Muscle, or Fat)

Identify Your Probable Type Class
(Thin, Muscle, or Fat)

———

Read the following three type classes: *Thin, Muscle and Fat,* and decide where you may fit. As you proceed to the individual body types within each class, the identity of your specific type becomes clearer. I hope that this book helps you towards that end.

———

<u>*The Thin Types Class*</u>
(Ectomorphs)

* *Review these descriptive items: 18 or more indicate you are probably a Thin type. How many apply to you?*

☐ Lean face, are youthful looking

☐ Slight and soft muscles (have low strength compared to the muscle types)

☐ Quiet and peaceful voice

- ☐ Generally have low strength or weight-lifting ability)

- ☐ Little fat stores, fat easily controlled (are never obese, or heavy like other classes)

- ☐ Slender, lean build; some *neurogenic* and *marasmic* males may be medium-sized and strong (with a muscle sub-type)

- ☐ Have solitary grieving (find peace alone, rather than share feelings with others)

- ☐ Most are concerned about health and aging (some neurotically so)

- ☐ Emotionally sensitive and sentimental

- ☐ Most only slight-moderate athletic ability (except some *marasmic and neurogenics*)

- ☐ Emotionally reserved (difficult to express deep emotions)

- ☐ Moderately passive and non-aggressive (except sillevitic)

- ☐ Low physical risk-taking (not dare-devils; discern risks before taking action)

- ☐ Not controlling (except for some sillevitics)

☐ Quick reaction times

☐ Tend to be insecure

☐ Need time for self in relationships

☐ Exercise not essential for health

☐ Mostly non-addicted*

☐ Generally introverted*

☐ Not impressive managers or leaders

☐ Are mostly self-conscious*

☐ Some socio-phobic; hard to relax socially*

☐ Most feel awkward in new situations*

☐ Have postural awareness

☐ Restrained verbal expression, tend to edit thoughts before speaking*

[* Exceptions — sillevitic and neurogenic types]

Total Checks = _____

More then 18 = <u>Probably</u> a Thin Type

If being a **Thin** *type seems probable to you,
read the brief descriptions of those types in
Chapter 2. If you do not identify with a* **Thin**
type description, note that certain **Muscle** *types
may be strong, but quite lean, particularly when
younger: the medeic, female myogenic,
nitropheric, and carbogenic types; see if you fit
there.*

*Good luck in finding   your body type, and in
attaining a greater degree of health and weight
control.*

The Muscle Types Class
(Mesomorphs)

* *Review these descriptive items: 16 or more indicate you are probably a Muscle type. How many apply to you?*

☐ Predominately strong bones and muscles

☐ Medium-build (some *medeic, myogenic, and nervimotives* may be lean like Thin types)

☐ Are naturally strong (and may attain great strength with body-building)

☐ Some are overly-sensitive

☐ Like to be in control (some excessively so)

☐ Outgoing and extroverted

☐ High physical courage ideal for combat

☐ Hard workers, industrious

☐ Are born leaders and managers

☐ Rarely obese; excess fat occurs after age 20-30 (mostly in *desmogenics and pallinomics*)

☐ Intelligent with some intellectuals

☐ High energy and vitality when healthy

- ☐ Motivation high, positively directed towards accomplishing goals
- ☐ Voice is strong, authoritative (many accomplished singers, actors)
- ☐ Prefer out-of-doors activities, enjoy nature
- ☐ Athletic, cream of Olympic medalists; need exercise for health
- ☐ Mostly have highly developed social values
- ☐ Mostly a positive attitude and persona
- ☐ Always ready to take action
- ☐ Good students (studious, accomplished; some hampered by drugs, boredom)
- ☐ Are mostly impassioned
- ☐ Have a temper, may anger easily
- ☐ Self-activating (accomplish goals)

Total Checks = _____

More then 16 = <u>Probably</u> Muscle Type

_____

———

*If being a **Muscle** type seems probable to you, read the brief descriptions of those types in Chapter 3. Note that certain **Muscle** types are strong, but may be quite lean and look like **Thin** types, particularly when younger: the medeic, female myogenic, nitropheric, and carbogenic types.*

*Also note that three **Fat** types, particularly when younger, may look like **Muscle** types: the oxyferic, isogenic, and pargenic types.*

Good luck in finding your body type, and in attaining a greater degree of health and weight control.

———

The Fat Types
(Endomorphs)

* *Review these descriptive items: 18 or more indicate you are probably a fat type. How many apply to you?*

☐ Fatty abdomen, upper arms and thighs

☐ Are physically expansive and strong

☐ Fat is gained progressively from early childhood (if not gained until after 20-30, then try *desmogenics and pallinomics*)

☐ Are usually happy and optimistic (in spite of weight)

☐ Mentally strong (may be intellectually powerful, brilliant)

☐ Learn from people and life; few are university-trained

☐ Receiving appreciation, affection, and approval are important

☐ Exercise not a priority (keys to weight control are willpower and diet)

☐ Reaction times are slow and methodical; nothing is done suddenly

☐ Good or superior business sense

- ☐ Radiate optimism, cheerfulness, and self-confidence

- ☐ Are even-tempered, calm and peaceful, but if upset are capable of 'raising the roof with outrage'

- ☐ Good digestion (an efficient and powerful digestive tract is typical, and it may be taxed to the limit!)

- ☐ Polite, considerate, generous, and giving of self to others

- ☐ Sleep deeply and may snore loudly; difficult to awaken

- ☐ Intelligent, many intellectuals

- ☐ Usually look fleshy, vulnerable to holding excessive fat, often from birth

- ☐ Assertive, some very aggressive

- ☐ More fun and pleasure loving than other type classes

- ☐ Love comfort and luxury (seek and often gain riches)

- ☐ Intensely love food (may be great cooks)

- ☐ Will-power weaker in most

☐ Voice made to be heard: it is strong, loud, assertive

☐ May have alcohol or substance abuse at some point in life (although rarely found drunk, or out-of-control)

Total Checks = _____

More then 19 = <u>*Probably*</u> *Fat Type*

————

If being a **Fat** *type seems probable to you, read the brief descriptions of those types in Chapter 4. Note that certain* **Muscle** *types may be quite fat when older: the desmogenic and pallinomic types.*

Good luck in finding your body type, and in attaining a greater degree of health and weight control.

————

2

Brief Descriptions:

The 6 Thin Types:

__Brief Descriptions__
Thin Types

Review these summaries to help identify your probable Thin type. Presented here are a few helpful celebrity examples (with many others provided throughout __The 22 Unique Body Types__ book).

▶ *Predominant "Yes" answers helps identify your type.*

———

The Atrophic Type

☐ Poorly absorb nutrients, deficiencies are common; very difficult to gain weight

☐ Usually thin, lean, gaunt, fragile

☐ Short or tall

☐ Weak bones, fragile health, physically weak

☐ Teeth, weak, white or gray, irregular

☐ Rosy cheeks often (mostly females)

☐ Mostly sensitive to altitude, barometrics

☐ Weak lungs, sinus, chronic infections

☐ Are passive, introverted, exclusive

☐ Intelligent, intellectual, debaters

☐ Born to be a vegetarian (or vegan)

☐ Pessimistic now, optimistic about the future

☐ Larger head, forehead, with a slight body

☐ Long face from large forehead to the chin

☐ Hair thin, oily

☐ Wide mouth, husky voice

☐ Skin moist, easily irritated

☐ Many health concerns throughout life

☐ Readily charm the opposite sex

☐ Many crave sex; moderately strong sex drive

☐ Strong will-power

☐ Most dislike physical labor (should not do it)

☐ May appear aloof, moody, bashful

☐ Enjoy solitude, being withdrawn

☐ May feel superior, disdainful, pessimistic

☐ Skeptical, some arrogant, unsociable

☐ Generally low faith in orthodox religions

Examples:

Woody Allen   *Audrey Hepburn*

Pee Wee Herman   *Calista Flockheart*

———

The Exesthesic Type

- [ ] A female-only rare type, oval face
- [ ] Desire cooked sulfur foods: cabbage, cauliflower, garlic, broccoli, etc.
- [ ] Are attractive or beautiful; feminine, have a lovely voice
- [ ] Appear slender and shapely with long legs
- [ ] Ethical, sincere, exclusive nature
- [ ] Trustworthy, responsible
- [ ] Are assertive, never passive
- [ ] Sensual: attract men like bees to honey
- [ ] May have angry episodes (or rage); tend to be unforgiving when wronged
- [ ] Authoritative, aggressive, prideful
- [ ] Are artistic and creative
- [ ] May be fussy, intense, impatient
- [ ] Usually honest, cultured, aristocratic
- [ ] Medium-sized or tall; medium to large bust
- [ ] Spine, tendons and joints easily stressed
- [ ] Eyelids vulnerable to irritation or infection

- ☐ Lovely skin, flush easily; little perspiration
- ☐ Aches and pains common (often on the left side of the body)
- ☐ Are creative, humorous, competent, optimistic
- ☐ Intelligent with some intellectuals
- ☐ Hard working, industrious, practical, good management ability
- ☐ More likely to be school cheer-leaders than athletes
- ☐ High self: confidence and image
- ☐ Tend to need sympathy
- ☐ Nervousness is very common
- ☐ Dislike: loud noises, electrical storms, heated rooms, cold
- ☐ Natural assertiveness may upset others
- ☐ Have domestic skills: home-making, etc.

Examples: (Female type only)
Cher   Sarah Jessica Parker

———

The Marasmic Type

☐ Always tall and lean, never short

☐ Some strong males (pro-athletes); are the strongest thin type

☐ Face is long, pleasant or attractive looking

☐ Prominent cheekbones, sunken cheeks

☐ Joints weaker, bones longer and stronger than most *Thin* types

☐ Some have deformed chest structure (males); smaller than average bust

☐ Males ruggedly handsome; females plain, pretty, rarely beautiful

☐ Voice authoritative, impressive

☐ Good leadership abilities, managers

☐ Honest, ethical, high integrity

☐ Quick learners, talented

☐ Creative and original thinkers

☐ Intelligent, may be brilliant; some intellectuals

☐ May be shy

☐ Some are reserved, sarcastic

☐ Some are stubborn, withdrawn

☐ May be distrustful, controlling, or aloof

☐ May be co-dependent, self-judgmental

☐ Some have addictive vulnerability (males)

☐ Have anxiety around opposite sex

☐ Have talent for teaching

☐ High self-confidence and self-image

☐ Females attractive, pretty

[Note – Some marasmics look like atrophics.]

Examples:
    Clint Eastwood   President George Bush, Sr.,
    Princess Diana   Vanessa Redgrave

———

The Neurogenic Type

☐ Are usually slender (or medium-build), short or tall

☐ Some men gain weight when older

☐ Small chest and bust (some moderate-sized)

☐ Lower jaw and chin smaller and narrower than average; may have wider jaw angles (due to *desmogenic or nervimotive* sub-type)

☐ Forehead often larger than average (particularly males)

☐ Large forehead may take up half the face; wide temples

☐ Thin hair, balding starts by age 20 (in males)

☐ Can talk all day, humorous (companions must be good listeners)

☐ Are quiet, mental, peaceful, creative, artistic, interesting

☐ Normal or small ears; some odd-shaped (particularly males)

☐ Some have neurotic tendency; may need, or have taken medication

☐ Tend to worry excessively; nervous, stressed

☐ Refined, cultured, aristocratic, nervous

☐ Are emotionally and physically sensitive, sentimental

☐ Often have unusual psychosomatic ailments (that confound doctors)

☐ Some males can weight-lift effectively; females weaker

☐ Blue or brown eyes; eyebrows thin, fine, high

☐ Relatively wide distance between eyebrows and eyes

☐ Intelligent, some intellectuals

☐ Hair is fine, thin; fair, brown or black

☐ Attracted to holistic healing, metaphysics

☐ Appear cultured (whether are or not)

☐ Have communication skills (singing, speaking, teaching)

Examples:
   President Dwight Eisenhower
   Ben Kinsley
   Jane Seymour   *Joan/Melissa Rivers*

The Pathoferic Type

☐ Are slender to medium-sized, average or moderately tall

☐ Smooth cheekbones, smaller chin

☐ Teen acne may occur into adulthood

☐ Small weak teeth (need cosmetic dentistry)

☐ Pleasant face, no cheekbone markings

☐ Are youthful, devoted, gentle, loving, creative

☐ Are mental, studious

☐ Self-conscious, sentimental

☐ Excessively forgiving, know no malice

☐ Dislike raising voice, may be co-dependent

☐ Have low assertiveness, no aggression

☐ Sedentary, withdrawn, high degree of modesty

☐ Strong God/spiritual belief, metaphysics

☐ Disgusted by aggression, raised voices, unkindness, violence

☐ Do not express anger (walk from arguments)

☐ Body slight to moderate, strong back and legs

- ☐ If female, are angelic; if male, women want you as a friend
- ☐ Muscles unresponsive to weight lifting
- ☐ Usually dislike hard physical work
- ☐ Often sickly when young, weak skin and lungs
- ☐ Overly accepting and forgiving of others
- ☐ Non-addicted to cigarettes, alcohol, drugs
- ☐ Emotionally withdrawn, many 'wall-flowers'
- ☐ Easily hurt; difficult to share emotional pain
- ☐ Tend to place others' feelings ahead of own
- ☐ In relationships, may be co-dependent
- ☐ Respect viewpoints of other people
- ☐ Lack management ability (but willing to try)
- ☐ May have low self-esteem and self-confidence
- ☐ If accused, are slow to respond
- ☐ May decline to defend self
- ☐ Humble, shy, slow to engage

Examples: (Celebrity examples are very rare)
Gwyneth Paltrow   Blythe Danner

———

The Sillevitic Type

☐ Usually thin, slender, medium-height or taller

☐ Have strong muscles and ligaments

☐ Are attractive or handsome

☐ Often blue-eyed, some brown

☐ Long face from forehead to chin

☐ If unhealthy, may have waxy rosy cheeks (females particularly)

☐ Hair fine, often fair, blonde, or brown, and lovely if healthy

☐ Sensitive lungs (or have had lung disease); may have smoked

☐ Some have weak or disfigured teeth; may need cosmetic dentistry

☐ Cluttered home, office and car is typical

☐ Enjoy public speaking, teaching, able to influence and inspire others

☐ Tend to suffer from excess self-importance and self-egotism

☐ Creative, metaphysical, expressive

☐ Optimistic, exclusive, positive, demeanor

☐ Are exotic, strong and often excessive ego

☐ Have difficulty living in the moment; always looking to tomorrow and the future

☐ Feel superior around peers (and often are)

☐ Always talking, honestly express opinions (can sell anything)

☐ Self-centered, tend to be critical, judgmental

☐ Idealistic, altruistic, desire to help mankind

☐ Excellent ability to socialize and converse with anyone: prince or pauper

☐ Happy, outgoing, optimistic, young looking

☐ Cravings, addictions are common: coffee, nicotine, alcohol, sugar, drugs, etc.

☐ Strong ego, assertive, aggressive (which may upset others)

☐ Often interested in new age healing, yoga and metaphysics

☐ Age gracefully (better than most types)

Examples:
David Bowie	*Rod Stewart*
Carol Burnett	*Carol Channing*

―――――

3

Brief Descriptions:

The 9 Muscle Types

Brief Descriptions:
Muscle Types

Review these summaries to help identify your probable Thin type. Presented here are a few helpful celebrity examples (with many others provided throughout The 22 Unique Body Types book).

▶ *A predominance of "Yes" answers helps identify your type.*

———

The Calciferic Type

☐ Are very rare, and potentially brilliant, esteemed, or famous

☐ Have an unmistakable commanding presence

☐ Are very tall, lean, medium-sized, heavier with age, and very strong

☐ Thin or balding hair in males is common (with aging)

☐ A powerful mind and intellect that is more powerful than other types

☐ Resilient, dedicated, tenacious, commanding

☐ Are scientific, original, creative, patient, friendly

☐ Tend to be slow, stern, stubborn, awkward, unyielding

☐ Are peaceful, but forceful or abusive if provoked

☐ Are the hardest workers; superior in leadership and intellect

☐ Great objectivity; do not rely on faith, trust, beliefs or sentiments; only interested in facts

☐ Voice is strong, urging, deep, forceful, emphatic, harsh, and abrupt

☐ Are plain looking or ruggedly attractive

☐ Powerful in debate; nobody thinks better on their feet than you do!

Examples:
  Daniel Day-Lewis Michael Jordan
  Angelica Huston Robin Wright

———

The Carbogenic Type

☐ Are all heights, medium-sized, strong body (particularly males)

☐ Are often handsome, attractive, beautiful or vivacious

☐ Hair growth usually plentiful; many males prematurely grey (often in their 20's)

☐ Males may have a hairy chest (or not, depending on sub-type)

☐ Females medium to large bust (depending on sub-type)

☐ Males often have a beard-line even after shaving (like *pargenics*)

☐ Are happy, cheerful, likable, charming, flirtatious

☐ Some vanity, particularly males

☐ Strong ego and abilities in career direction

☐ High self-confidence (more than most types)

☐ High intelligence, some intellectuals

☐ Peace-loving, highly social and conversational

☐ Some males are macho or misogenists

☐ May be co-dependent when younger

☐ Many are sensual and/or sexual, with a strong sex drive

☐ Attract the opposite sex like bees to honey

☐ Exude a sensuality that the opposite sex finds hard to resist

☐ Some have a weak conscience, and low will-power

☐ May become moody if not getting their own way

Examples:
Alec Baldwin   Mel Gibson
Lady Gaga
Lora Logan ("60 Minutes")

———

The Desmogenic Type

☐ Very strong muscles and tendons

☐ Lean and wiry when young (often heavier with age)

☐ Have high intelligence, some intellectuals

☐ Are aggressive leaders with a commanding presence

☐ Have genuine courage; fearless in the face of the enemy

☐ Speak your mind very bluntly and honestly

☐ Bold and big risk-takers (hence are big successes or failures)

☐ Ambitious for power and leadership (and usually achieve it)

☐ Think, feel, and act with conviction and intensity

☐ Prominent cheek bones, sunken cheeks; a muscular wide chin

☐ Many singers; voice is strong, resilient; musical talents

☐ Pointed angles of jaw (markedly in men; less-so in females)

☐ Emotional intensity and passions creates relationship problems

☐ Highly sensual, an intense sex drive often from early childhood

☐ Some are moody, combative, controlling, intimidating

☐ Non-magnetic personality, rule by domination and coercion

☐ Desire to be in control or in command

☐ Dimpled chin common in males (and some other muscle types)

☐ Balding tendency common (most bald males are this type or *neurogenic*)

☐ Females often beautiful; males attractive or ruggedly handsome

☐ Joint pain or arthritis common with age

☐ Forcefully and fearlessly express opinions

Examples:
   Daniel Craig   Val Kilmer
   Loni Anderson
   Madeleine Albright (Sec. of State),

———

The Eldic Type

☐ Are often <u>shorter</u> than average (or medium-height); never tall

☐ Are attractive or handsome; often long-living, healthy and strong

☐ Lean to medium-sized shapely body, some heavier females

☐ Strong ideals, desire to help the planet, ecology or mankind

☐ Are honest, ethical, principled, honorable

☐ Invariably nice, pleasant, and happy

☐ Lower lip may be thin, taunt, and flat

☐ Ears larger than normal in males; females more average-sized

☐ Males may look tough and wiry; ruggedly handsome

☐ Females are, or were, tom-boys (tend to dislike wearing skirts)

☐ Some freckled and red-headed; abundant hair growth for life

☐ Vertical lines around a wider mouth (males particularly)

☐ With aging may have a lined face (more than other types)

☐ Are sincere, pleasant, honest, responsible

☐ Some highly sensual, others not

☐ Have technical skills and abilities (both sexes)

☐ Good and fair managers and leaders

☐ Moral, refined, ethical, charming, social

☐ Spiritual, honorable, strongly principled

☐ Highly intelligent with some intellectuals

☐ Some stubborn and unreasonably obstinate

Examples:
Dustin Hoffman   *William H. Macy*
Hillary Rodham Clinton
Shirley MacLaine

———

The Medeic Type

☐ Have a lean to medium-sized body (some thin or gaunt, but strong)

☐ Tend to be wiry, plain, homely

☐ Are intelligent or intellectual

☐ Males have little or no body hair

☐ Rugged beauty or attractiveness when young, more plain with age

☐ Many are highly creative with a dramatic and tragic sense

☐ May be stern, angry, intense, aggressive

☐ May be sexually demanding with high cravings

☐ You may have unusual social and sexual mores

☐ Male chest has little body hair; bust usually small to medium-sized (some large depending on their sub-type)

☐ Nose small and squat, sometimes larger; nose-tip may be long

☐ Muscles small and compact, very strong

☐ If offended, are quick to punish

☐ Often gesticulate when talking

☐ May be overly-familiar, or antisocial

☐ Difficult to gain weight

☐ Have great tenacity; very excitable and restless

☐ Excessively strict, some liberal

☐ Personality may have a dark side; desire alcohol, pot, etc.

☐ May look older than they are

Examples:

David Caruso	*Humphrey Bogart*
Madonna	*Sandra Bernhard*

———

The Myogenic Type

☐ Are eloquent and personable

☐ Usually slender to medium, muscular, may gain weight with age

☐ Medium height or tall, handsome, attractive, or beautiful

☐ Have athletic potential, youthful

☐ Idealistic, intelligent

☐ Are bright, some brilliant and intellectual

☐ Are positive, friendly, action-oriented

☐ Are leaders, motivators, born managers

☐ Are congenial, optimistic

☐ Love nature, full of life

☐ Love social communion

☐ Assess risks and are brave, fearless, and courageous (highly decorated in war-time)

☐ Out-going, romantic, and influential

☐ Some have moral and willpower weakness

☐ Low impulse control is common: sex, drugs, etc. (as in Presidents Kennedy and Clinton)

☐ Hair is full, thick in males: fine, wavy in females; all colors; usually maintain growth throughout life (unless have a bald sub-type)

☐ Natural managers, organizers, and planners

☐ Idealistic, unselfish, giving of themselves

☐ Happy, outgoing, optimistic

☐ Tolerant of other people's opinions, able to maintain poise in chaotic situations

☐ Empathetic and sympathetic to others' feelings (to a fault)

☐ Able to express self eloquently

☐ Able to stubbornly defend your point of view

☐ Are very bright, some esteemed scholars (Pres. Bill Clinton)

☐ Strong prominent muscles in males, lean and strong females (many Olympic athletes)

☐ Desire in some way to help mankind, planet

☐ Enjoy influencing others: teaching, speaking, advising, etc.

Examples:
  Robert Redford   *President Bill Clinton*
  Julia Roberts   *Jacqueline Onassis*

———

The Nervimotive Type

☐ Males are strong and attractive; women are pretty or lovely

☐ Nose usually small, snub or thin; some large

☐ Lungs large, strong

☐ Face often wide at cheekbones

☐ Vertical lines in cheeks are common

☐ Wide lower jaw at ears; jaw line may slope straight to chin

☐ Upper lip often thin; lower lip variable

☐ Are high-tempered, intolerant of fools

☐ Are often long-living

☐ Are rational, practical, gifted, and artistic

☐ Have high values and ethics

☐ May be demanding, suspicious, accusative

☐ Many are hard working, brilliant,intellectual

☐ Usually fiery, nervous, passionate, volatile

☐ Give 110% until drop from exhaustion

☐ Attracted to learning, power, education, reputation, position

☐ Male chest often hairy; medium or large bust

☐ Impassioned, strong ideals, fight for a cause

☐ Dark, brunette lovely hair that grays early

☐ Hairline straight across the forehead; widow peak is common

☐ Tend to know-it-all: want others to accept their views

☐ May have awkward jerky movements; some part of the body may always be moving (particularly in males)

☐ Square-rectangular forehead; may show vertical forehead profile

☐ May be mystical and intuitive

☐ Have good business judgment

☐ Highly impassioned, strongly idealist, fight for a cause

☐ Excellent ability to socialize and converse with people

Examples:
Jack Nicholson   *Frank Sinatra*
Elizabeth Taylor   *Natalie Wood*

———

The Nitropheric Type

☐ Are medium-height or tall

☐ Handsome, attractive, or beautiful

☐ Teeth white, strong, shapely, attractive

☐ Are leaders, intelligent with some intellectuals

☐ Sensitive to injustice and false accusation

☐ Passive and tranquil until hidden feelings are explosively expressed

☐ *Males*: sparse or slight chest hair (some exceptions); are charming, rational, but some are chauvinistic or macho

☐ *Females*: medium to large bust; elegant and sophisticated; sentimental

☐ Other women are competitive or jealous of your feminine beauty

☐ Female decisions based on feelings (need more rational thinking)

☐ Live in the past; are romantic and sentimental

☐ Are physically and emotionally sensitive

☐ Deepest feelings are hidden

☐ Allow no compromise to ethics, moral compass or spirituality

☐ Able to take command; like being in-control

☐ Vulnerable to health problems from environmental toxicity

☐ Strong rivalry and jealousy sense; often excessively outspoken

☐ Tend to easily forgive and excuse own negative behaviors

☐ If offended you show calm, but the offender will probably pay

☐ Tardy tendency, keep others waiting; will not be rushed

☐ Show 'humanitarian' lines on forehead; females show fine lines

☐ Mouth and lips shapely or lovely; upper lip larger in the center

☐ Have an excellent ability to influence others

☐ Deep love feelings hidden, hard to express

☐ Appear serene, unruffled, poised, even if not

☐ Attractive cheeks, forehead square, rectangular

Examples:

Gregory Peck   *Ben Affleck*

Marilyn Monroe   *Jessica Lange*

―――――

The Pallinomic Type

☐ Rocine: "…are the most practical of all types"

☐ Are tall, strong, large, and muscular

☐ May be charming, desirable to opposite sex

☐ Medium-sized when young (gain fat after 25)

☐ Are leaders, modest, reserved;

☐ Intelligent and hard-working

☐ Are highly practical, self-actualizing, positive, optimistic, and successful

☐ Effective managers and supervisors

☐ Tend to be aggressive, willful, skeptical

☐ Are plain-speaking, impatient, sometimes unforgiving if ignored

☐ Are honest, plain-speaking (some are arrogant)

☐ Hair is often black, red, or wiry, and strong

☐ Are unimpressed by threats and don't back down from anyone

☐ Dislike immorality and crudeness; do not tolerate fools

☐ Are rational thinkers, some academics; learn wisdom from life

☐ High common sense, hate inactivity, enjoy hard physical work

☐ Are impressed by honest and self-controlled people

☐ Employees appreciate your intelligence and positive work-ethic

☐ Are not moved by tears and emotions; expect obedience to their will

Examples:
    President Donald Trump   *John Wayne*
    Att. Gen. Janet Reno   *Jane Russell*

———

4

Brief Descriptions:

The 7 Fat Types

Fat Types
Brief Descriptions

Review these summaries to help identify your probable Thin type. Presented here are a few helpful celebrity examples (with many others provided throughout The 22 Unique Body Types book).

▶ *A predominance of "Yes" answers helps identify your type.*

The Barotic Type

☐ Heavy, all heights, physically and mentally strong

☐ Large bony, broad body and abdomen (flat abdomen if not obese)

☐ Masculine body (both sexes); sexual expression not a priority

☐ Are usually calm, quite, humble, withdrawn, friendly, honest

☐ Are passive, serious, philosophical, practical, moral, ethical

☐ Appear timid (but are not); difficult to express deep feelings

☐ Are plain-speaking, peace-loving, genuine humility, humane

☐ Are slow to act, but dynamic when motivated or in emergencies

☐ Are intelligent with many intellectuals found

☐ Excellent ability to socialize and converse with anyone

☐ Impossible to kill or go to war

☐ Appear timid but are brave as lions if necessary

☐ Make life-long friends; are warm, sociable, interested, loyal

☐ Philosophers, love nature, the universe; are naturalists

Examples:
Robin Williams
Robin as "Mrs. Doubtfire"
(No female examples)

———

The Carboferic Type

☐ You are physically strong, all heights

☐ Are sensual, highly sexual; high level of jealousy

☐ Usually obviously fat as a child, may be obese later in life

☐ Some are medium-sized when younger, but heavier by age 20

☐ Fatty hips, abdomen; usually a large stomach

☐ Heavy upper arms, thin wrists, small hands and feet

☐ Are vivacious, magnetic, cheerful, friendly

☐ Are peaceful and peace-makers

☐ Mostly have *supreme* self-confidence (some males egocentric)

☐ May have some addictive tendencies

☐ Are social, engaging, and conversational

☐ Males often develop a bald spot starting in the back-head

☐ Are intelligent with many intellectuals found

☐ Generally not suited for the military or police (too lenient)

☐ Have music appreciation (playing, singing, performing, writing, etc.)

☐ Tend to be lazy and procrastinating

☐ Not good in an emergency (unlike the *barotic*)

☐ Outgoing personality, friendly

☐ Short distance between eyes and mouth (like the *hydripheric,* unlike the *isogenic)*

☐ Not a strong or forceful personality

Examples:
   Billy Gardell & Melissa McCarthy
   John Arnold   Roseanne Barr

———

The Hydripheric Type

☐ You are always heavy from early childhood

☐ Strong water-holding tendency (may slosh around in your tissues)

☐ Appear water-logged, physically weak and slow moving

☐ May look similar to *lipopherics* (but their fat is solid)

☐ Short distance eyes to mouth (like *carboferic*, unlike *isogenic*)

☐ Large and heavy lower face

☐ Are fat or obese, weight loss is very difficult

☐ Head narrow and flat, side to side, box-like appearance

☐ Short and thick lower legs and ankles; hands and feet small

☐ Joints weak, vulnerable, little strength for sports

☐ Large chest, pendulous bust is typical

☐ Peace lovers (angry war-talk means nothing), do not smile much

☐ High intelligence, with some intellectuals

- ☐ Mostly loving, serious, gentle, social, humorous, kind, and friendly
- ☐ Some are detached, disinterested, argumentative, belligerent
- ☐ Readily gain or lose ten pounds of water per week (and/or daily!)
- ☐ High sense of love, honor, kindness, peace, strife, disdain of war
- ☐ Sexual passion is strong and monogamous, have strong jealous sense
- ☐ May cry easily, but always in private (mainly females)
- ☐ Some may enter an unconscious hypnotic-like state for no reason!

Examples:
    Brian Dennehy   *Rodney Dangerfield*
    'Momma' Cass - 60's
    (Few female examples.)

———

The Isogenic Type

☐ Generally, males are never tall, females never short

☐ Shorter extremities make you taller on sitting, and shorter on standing

☐ Are medium-sized when younger.

☐ After age 30-35, females often gain weight (or become obese)

☐ While young, males are lean, some weight gain by middle-age

☐ Have a long and wide face; maintain a full head of hair

☐ Distance from eyes to mouth long (compared to *carboferic, hydripheric*)

☐ Strong sex drive

☐ Many are shy, honest, artistic, philosophical, idealistic, ethical

☐ May have 'wishy-washy' behaviors

☐ Slow learners, but may be brilliant, intelligent or intellectual

☐ Hands are short, square, hard, bony

☐ May be vulnerable to addiction (some are lazy, low achievers)

☐ Lymphatics are often a key health problem by causing lowering immunity

☐ Talk easily, have a loud voice, are fine teachers

☐ History of acne common (boils common in unhealthy males)

☐ Strong wedge-shape from shoulders to feet; hips; wide waist

☐ Are self-made: powerful mind and intellect (but may be lazy)

☐ Understand principles and natural laws easily

☐ May be brilliant; or prefer doing nothing, procrastinating, etc.

Examples:
    Phillip Seymour Hoffman   *Einstein*
    Oprah Winfrey   *Shelly Winters*

———

The Lipopheric Type

☐ Potentially the fattest of all types

☐ You are short or tall, and heavy or obese

☐ You often have large lips; are physically and mentally strong

☐ Large chest (medium-hairy in males); often a very large bust

☐ Relatively small top-head (heavy and large lower back-head)

☐ Dark or brown hair; a bald spot later appears at back-head

☐ A broad chin, deep dimple; usually double or triple chins

☐ Arms often quite hairy; the wrists are fatty, small hands

☐ Protruding fat abdomen in teens; fat ball in the cheeks

☐ You have a loud voice: friendly, outgoing, confident, pleasant

☐ Express carefully thought-out opinions, are naturally aggressive

☐ Are highly social, ego-centric, controlling, high intelligence

☐ Desire to serve others, plain-speaking, great communicators

☐ Some battle addictions; seek or have found God

☐ Mostly polite, happy, optimistic, humorous

☐ Show best side to strangers; very generous when have money

☐ Highly sentimental, love nature and 'the good life'

☐ Excellent salesmen; stretch the truth easily; sell anything to anyone!

☐ Able to scold and discipline others without anger or meanness

☐ Emphatic gestures of head and hands when communicating

☐ Producers, communicators, collaborators, activists, do-ers!

Examples:
Governor Chris Christie, Rush Limbaugh
Ricki Lake (few female examples)

———

The Oxypheric Type

☐ Are barrel-chested, heavy, medium-height or tall

☐ Medium-weight and size until young adults; later heavy or obese

☐ Large, bony, strong, florid face

☐ Head and face are large, smooth, impressive, no sharp edges

☐ Abdomen larger with age (particularly males)

☐ Handsome, attractive, brilliant, creative, charming, ambitious

☐ Altruistic, philosophical, communicators

☐ High intelligence, many intellectuals; strong belief in a God

☐ May be demanding, rebellious, aggressive, forcefully outspoken

☐ May be addicted to alcohol or drugs; tend to be epicurean

☐ After a few hours sleep, are recharged and ready to work again

☐ Flirtatious, charming, successful orators, public speakers or singers

☐ Practical, business oriented, active gestures

- ☐ Enjoy communicating with interesting people; 'do not suffer fools gladly'

- ☐ Out-going, exuberant, impulsive, and energetic; have bravado

- ☐ Are respected and admired by friends and enemies

- ☐ Are climactic: rise to the heights, then may fall, only to rise again

- ☐ May be overly-familiar; readily reveal deep thoughts, feelings

- ☐ Are engineers, capitalists, executives, entrepreneurs, authors, leaders

- ☐ Can talk to anyone, aristocratic

- ☐ High self-confidence and self-image are hallmarks of persona

Examples:
William Randolph Hearst
Orsen Wells
Ella Fitzgerald
Karita Mattila (many opera divas)

———

The Pargenic Type

☐ Medium-sized body when young; hold fat with aging

☐ Jet-black hair (some brown); age 30-40 start thinning or balding

☐ Brown, dark eyes typical; eyebrows, eyelashes stiff and sparse

☐ Nose may be larger than normal (some have a shiny nose-tip)

☐ Face may be fleshy (potential fatty), pock-marked, or acne-scarred

☐ A heavy lower jaw and double chin is common

☐ Upper lip is normal; lower lip may be loose, thicker and blue-red

☐ Teeth may be irregular, white or yellowing, and fragile

☐ Are sensual, expressive, with a serious and honest manner

☐ Intellectual, may be brilliant, powerful intellect, high intelligence

☐ High sex drive; may be sensuous

- ☐ Talented, hard working, serious, secretive, magnetic
- ☐ Some conceited, awkward, suspicious, untrusting, macho
- ☐ Are plain-speaking, ego-centric, may desire adulation
- ☐ Great reasoning power (many lawyers); do not appease anyone
- ☐ Some caustic, critical, argumentative, law unto themselves (Nixon)
- ☐ Willpower very strong, brave, daring, some may be conceited
- ☐ Some are antisocial, haughty
- ☐ Skin often irregular, lumpy or scarred, flaky, odorous, oily
- ☐ May tend to clandestine, conspiracy theories
- ☐ Some may be sociopathic, or need medication

> *Examples:*
> *President Nixon*   *Burt Reynolds*
> *Kirstey Alley*   *Katey Segal*

———

Summary

The brief descriptions of the 22 body types have given you a glimpse of your type. You may find it difficult to differentiate some of these types until you read the detailed descriptions in *The 22 Unique Body Types*. Note that keys to identifying the Fat types may be the personality aspects and celebrity examples.

———

5

Obtain your Detailed Type Data

Obtain your Detailed Type Data

Having identified your probable body type, order from the usual on-line source either your type booklet or for all body types *The 22 Unique Body Types*.

Your type data contains: all of the type descriptions and specific nutritional and dietary needs for health and weight loss, along with information on your health challenges, stress management, success spheres, spiritual challenges, personality strengths and weaknesses, and more…

Or if you prefer, refer to Appendix B for information on having Dr. Stenbeck help with your body type or those health-related issues amenable to an on-line consult.

———

Appendix

A. *Help Identify your Body Type with Dr. Stenbeck*

B. *On-line Health Consultation with Dr. Stenbeck*

Appendix A

Help Identify your Body Type With Dr. Stenbeck

If you desire help in identifying your body type, follow these instructions and answer the questionnaire. For further information and fees, send me an email from page one of the website:

DrStenbeck.net

First name: _____

Country of birth: _____

Upload photos and send to the above website:

- Head and shoulders: front and side views

- Full body: front and side views

- Also 1-2 teenage views

- If possible, casual photos of mother, father, siblings

MY TYPE CLASS MAY BE: _____

(Thin, Muscle, or Fat)

AGE   -   _____

HEIGHT   -   _____ feet/inches

MY WEIGHT -   _____ pounds

- Heaviest at age: _____

   - Lightest as adult: _____

   - Estimate age 15: _____

VISION - Excellent   Average   Poor:

HAIR -   Natural color: _____

   - Thin/thick? _____

   - balding? _____

SKIN - Quality: _____

   - History of acne, boils, other:

_____

_____

TEETH -   Strong   Weak   Dentures

 - Cavity history: Many   Moderate   Few

MUSCLES   -   Strong Average   Weak

    Sports played _____

JOINTS -   Strong   Average   Weak

HEALTH - Childhood diseases?

_____

_____

   - Adult diseases?

_____

AVERAGE DIET

     - Beef   _____ (times/week)

- Poultry   _____ (times/week)

- Fish   _____ (times/week)

- Eggs   _____ (times/week)

- Water   _____ (glasses/day):

- Vegetarian? Vegan?   _____

- Other?   _____

- Did your childhood diet differ? _____

The above will help me know who you are! I will send you a follow-up questionnaire for further help in identifying your body type.

Appendix B

On-line Health Consultation with Dr. Stenbeck

For further information, or to comment on this book, or to receive a response on any health issue from a holistic viewpoint, send an email inquiry from page one of my website:

DrStenbeck.net

Following that, I will suggest further healing needs, which we may pursue with an on-line consult.

———